# WHY DID I WORRY ABOUT THAT?

Written by Lyndsey Griffin-Cowap

Illustrated by Mark Lloyd

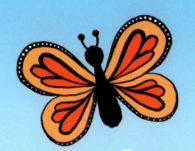
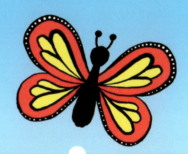

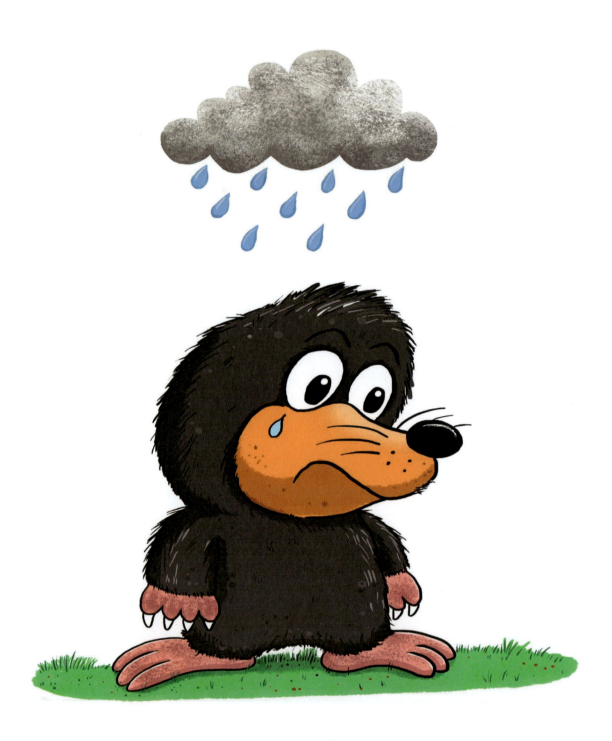

Once upon a time, there was a very worried mole called Monty. All he did was worry.

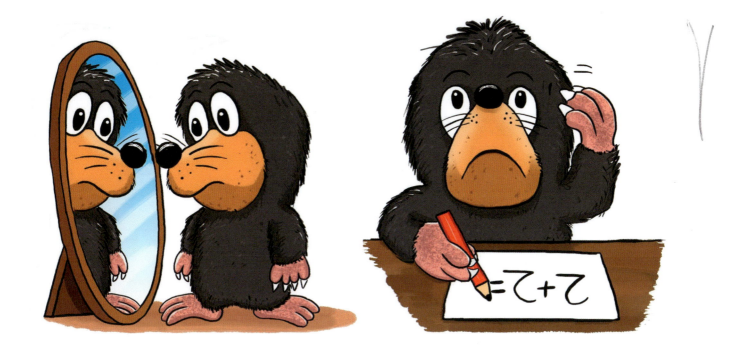

He worried that he did not look good.

He worried that he would not be able to do his school work.

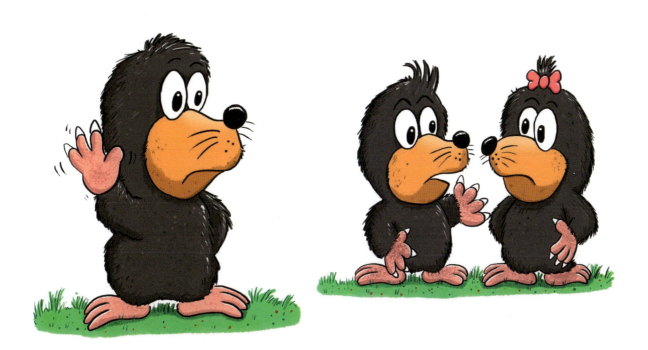

He worried that nobody would like him.

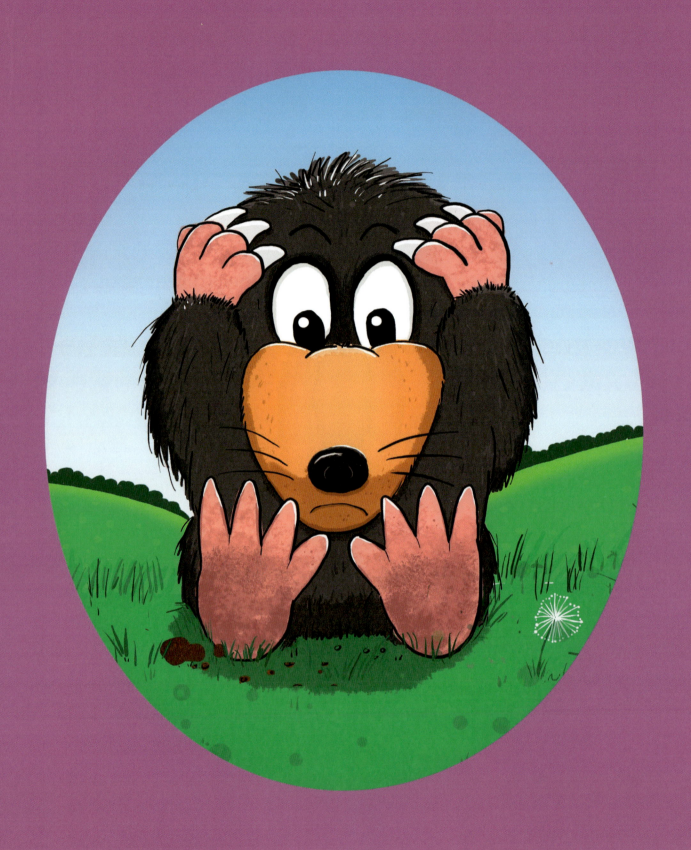

In fact, he worried when he had nothing to worry about, or when things had not even happened yet.

Every time he worried, he would roll up in a ball and bury his head in his hands.

Suddenly, Monty Mole heard a voice coming from the tree. It was his friend the Wise Old Owl.

"WHAT'S TO DO, WHAT'S TO DO, TOOWIT TOOWOO."

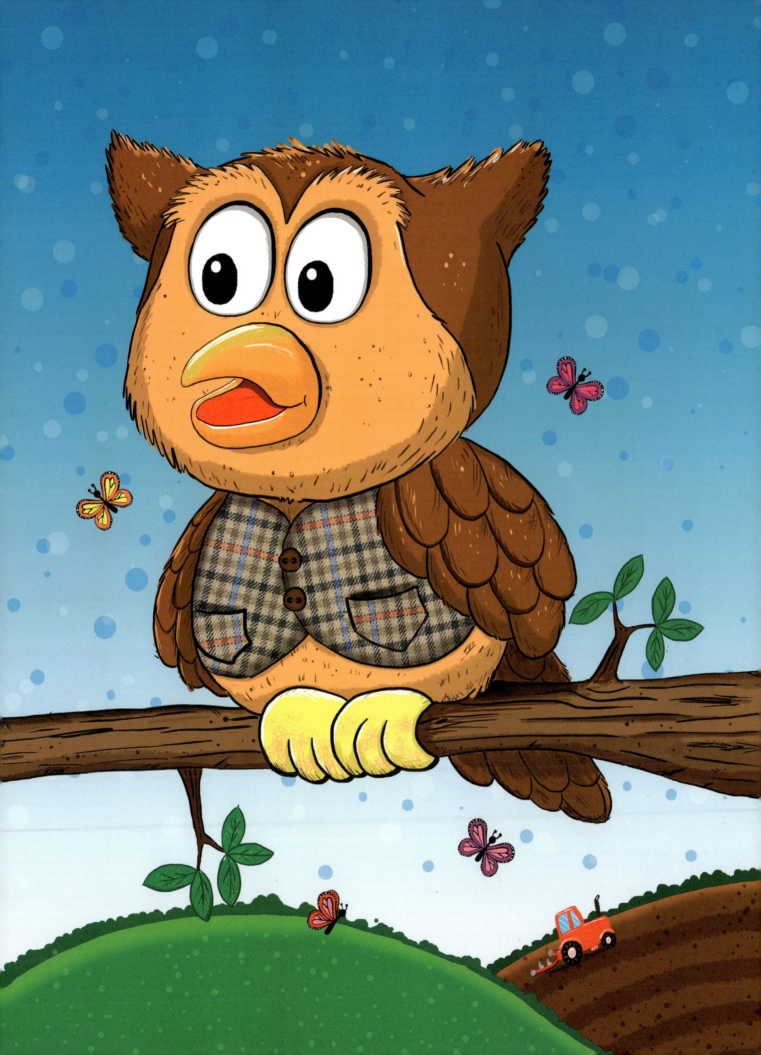

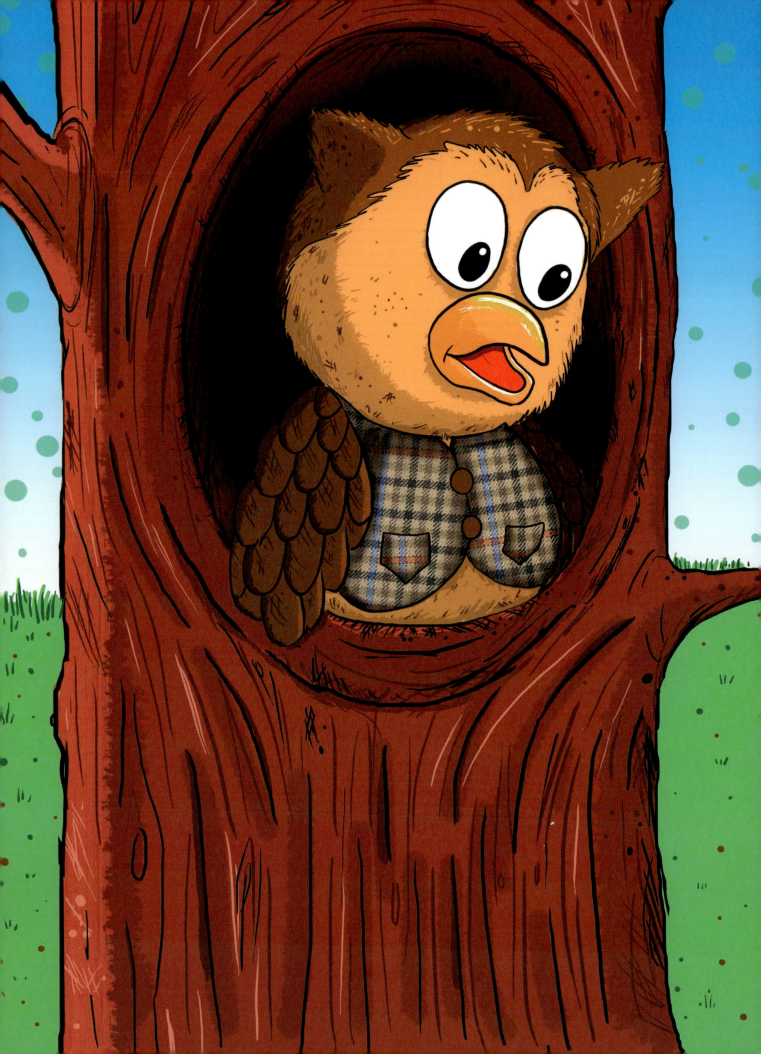

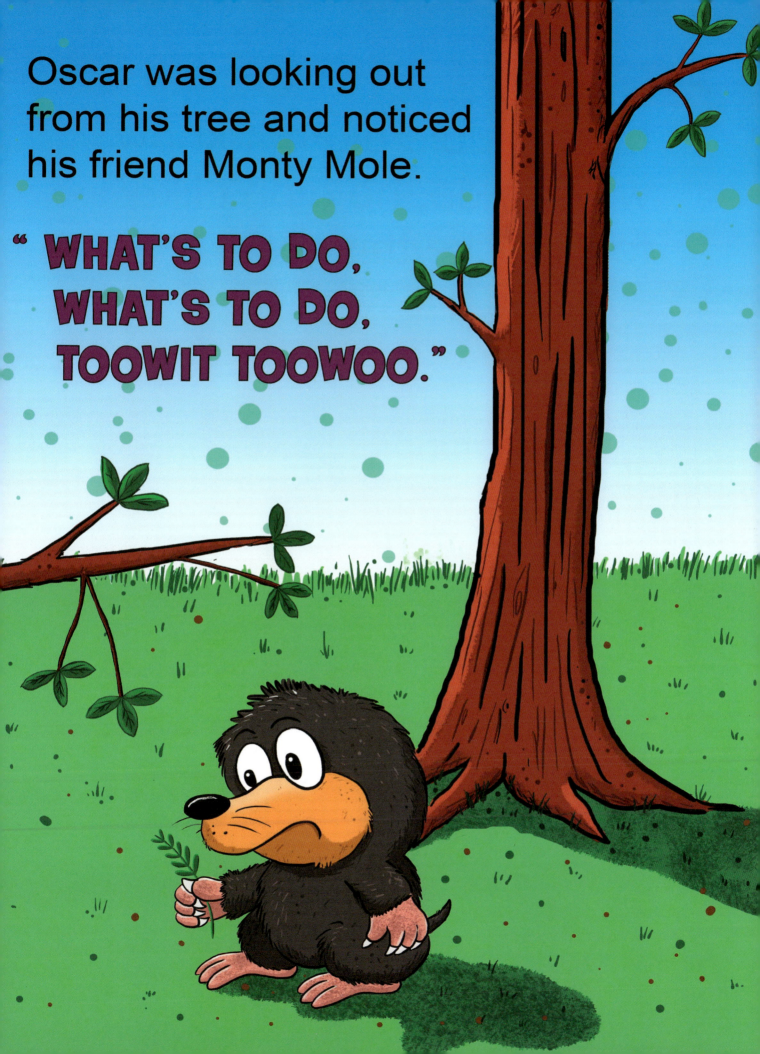

Monty Mole did not know what to do, he didn't like feeling like this.

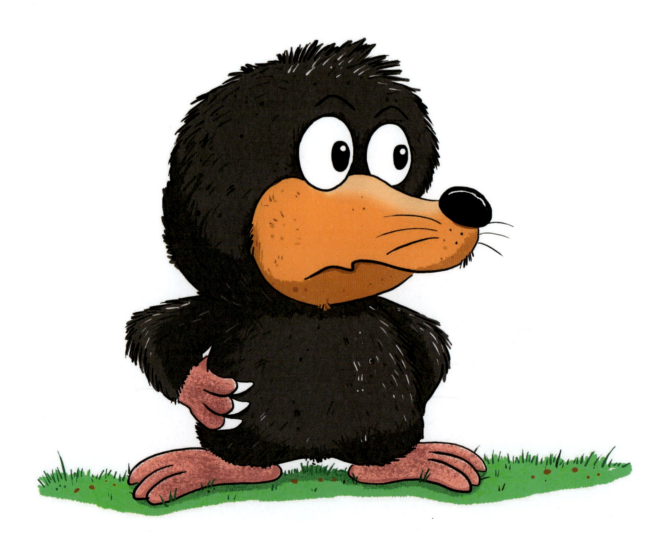

So Oscar the Owl thought for a while and then said "I've come up with a plan for you."

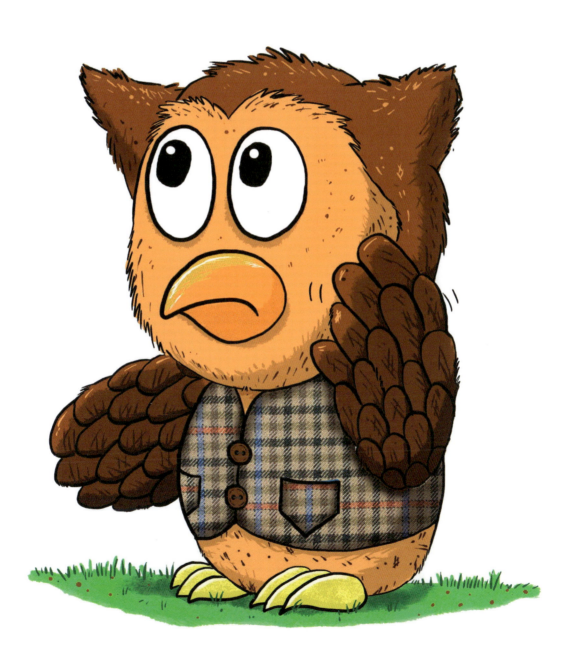

Let me introduce you to my box of butterflies.

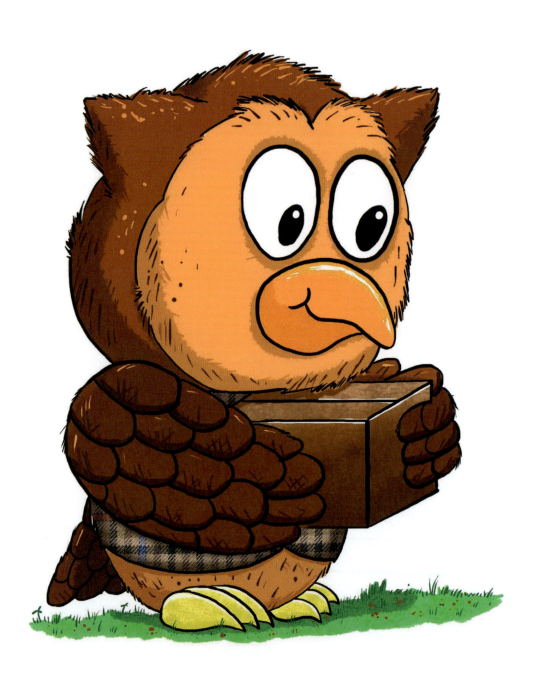

"That's funny," said Monty Mole, "I feel like I have butterflies in my tummy sometimes."

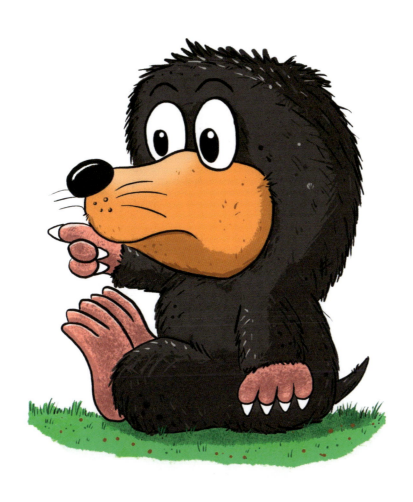

Nobody likes me

I don't look very nice

I can't do my school work

If you draw and write down all of your worries on some paper, or whisper your worries to the butterflies, you will soon begin to feel better.

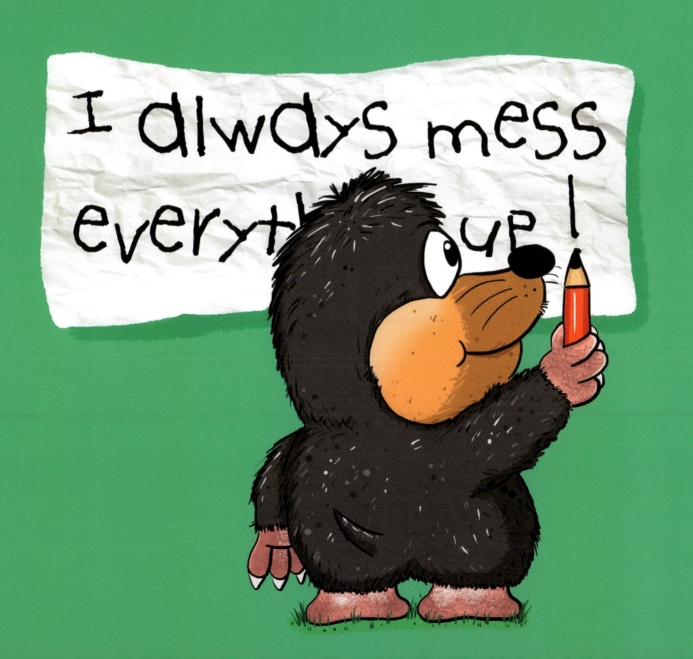

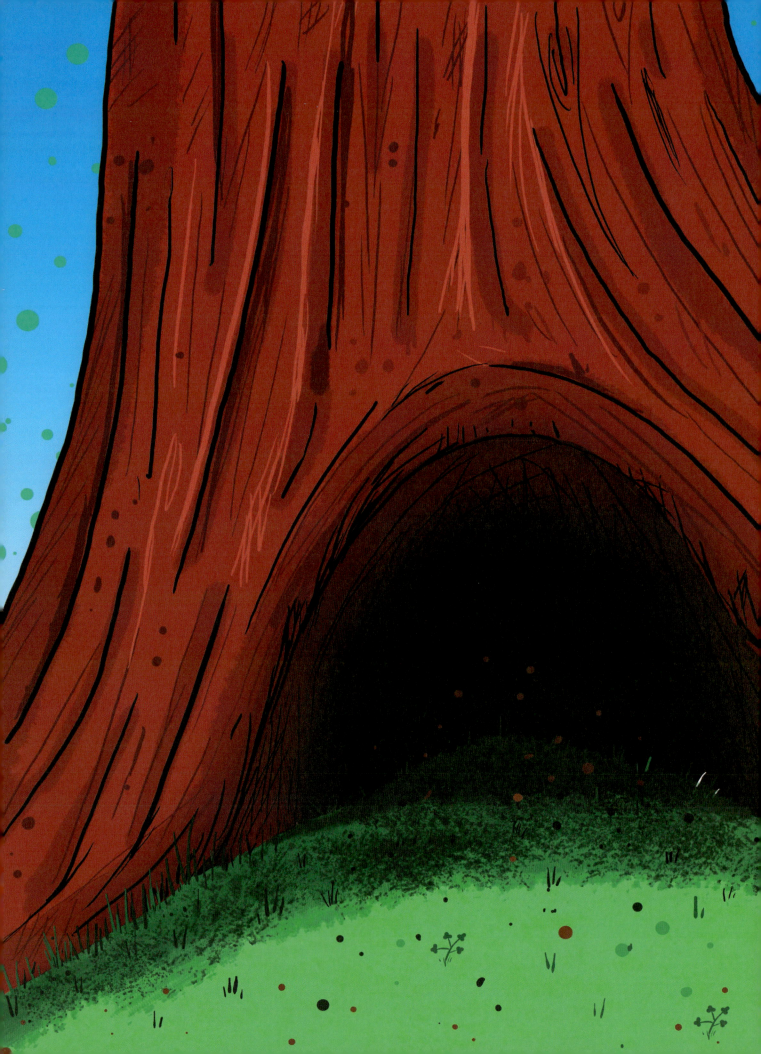

Oscar explained to Monty Mole, that if Monty took the box of butterflies to the nook of his tree, he would look after them.

"I will take care of them for you and those big worries will gradually shrink and some of the butterflies may even fly away".

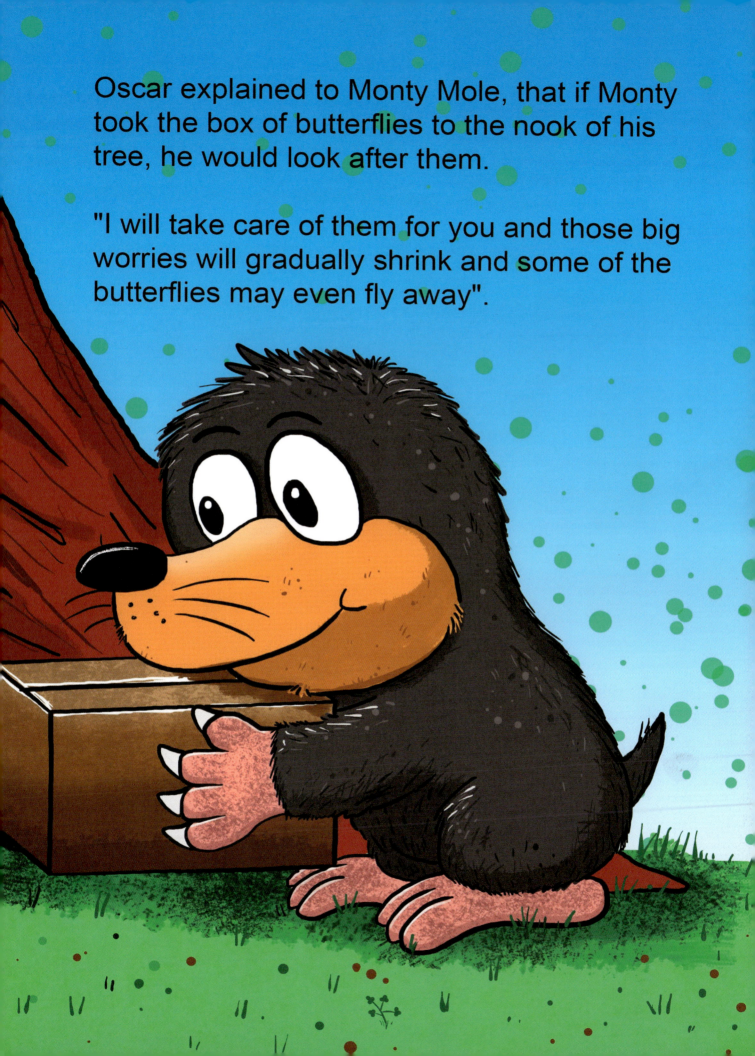

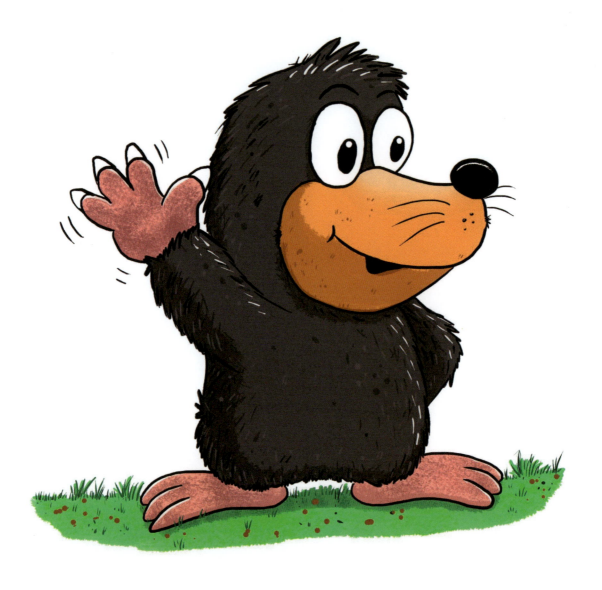

Monty Mole soon began to feel happier about himself and he realised that everyone did like him.

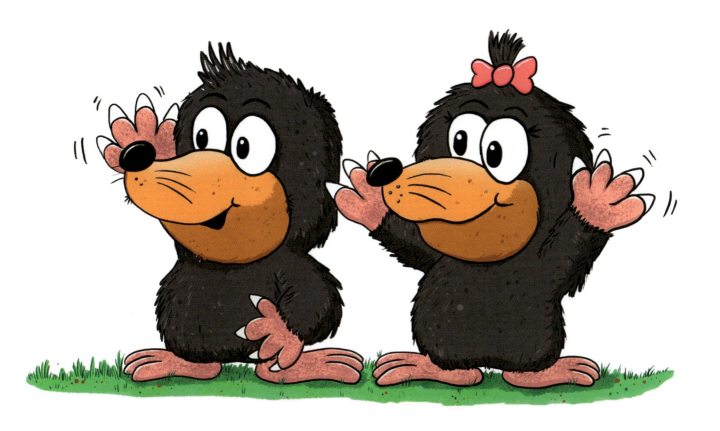

He was also able to do his school work and felt happier about the way he looked.

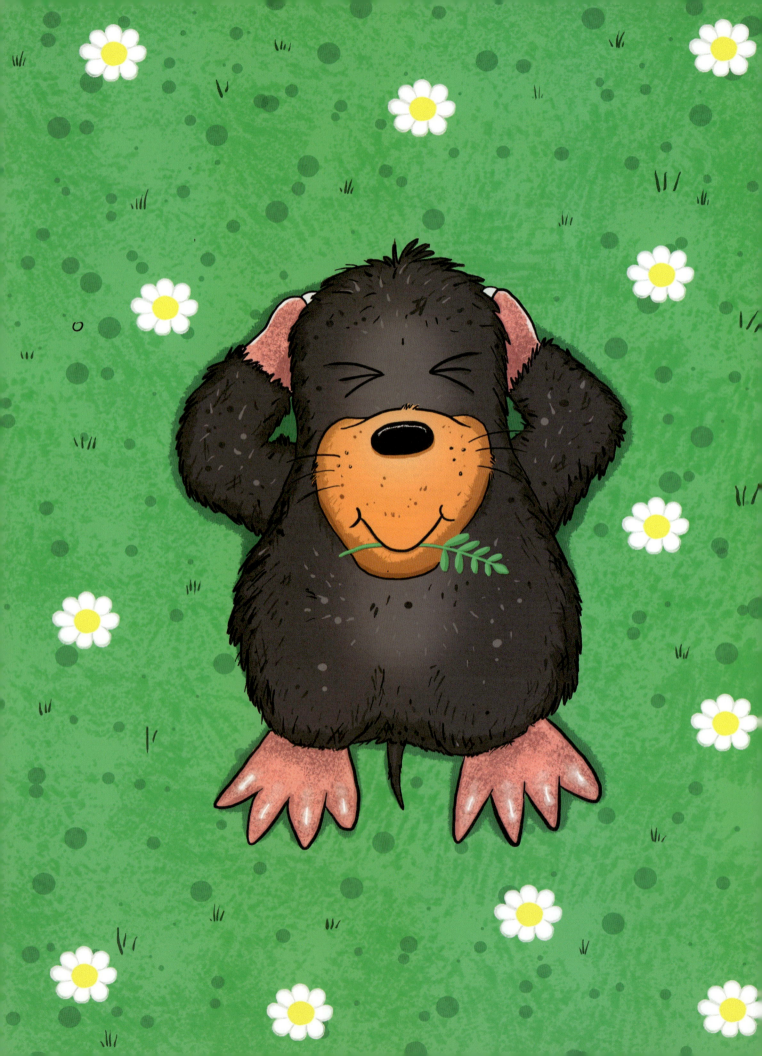

Monty Mole began to understand how to relax and cope with some of his worries.

Monty Mole started
to believe in himself
and he began to feel
happier.

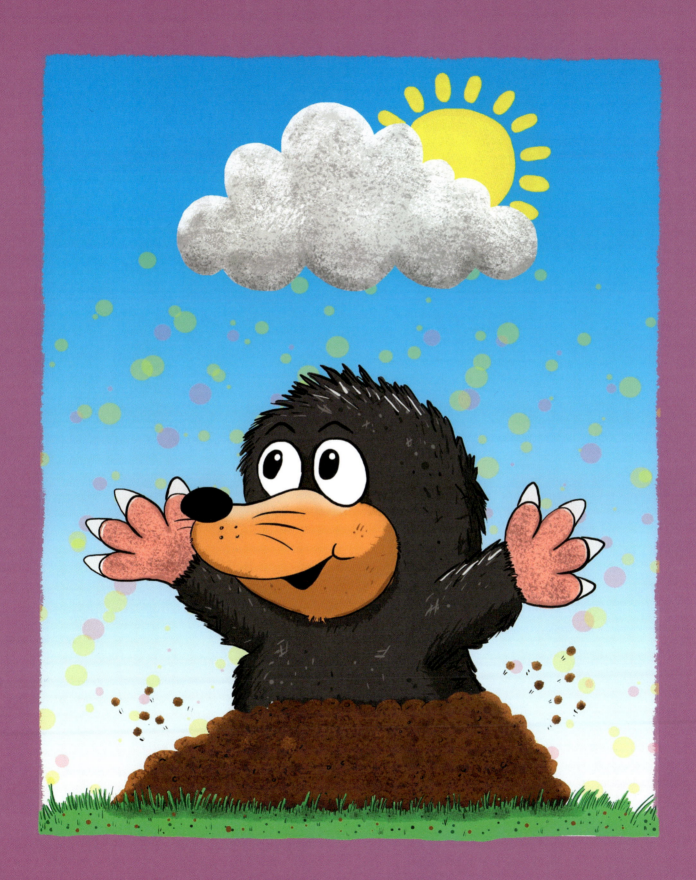

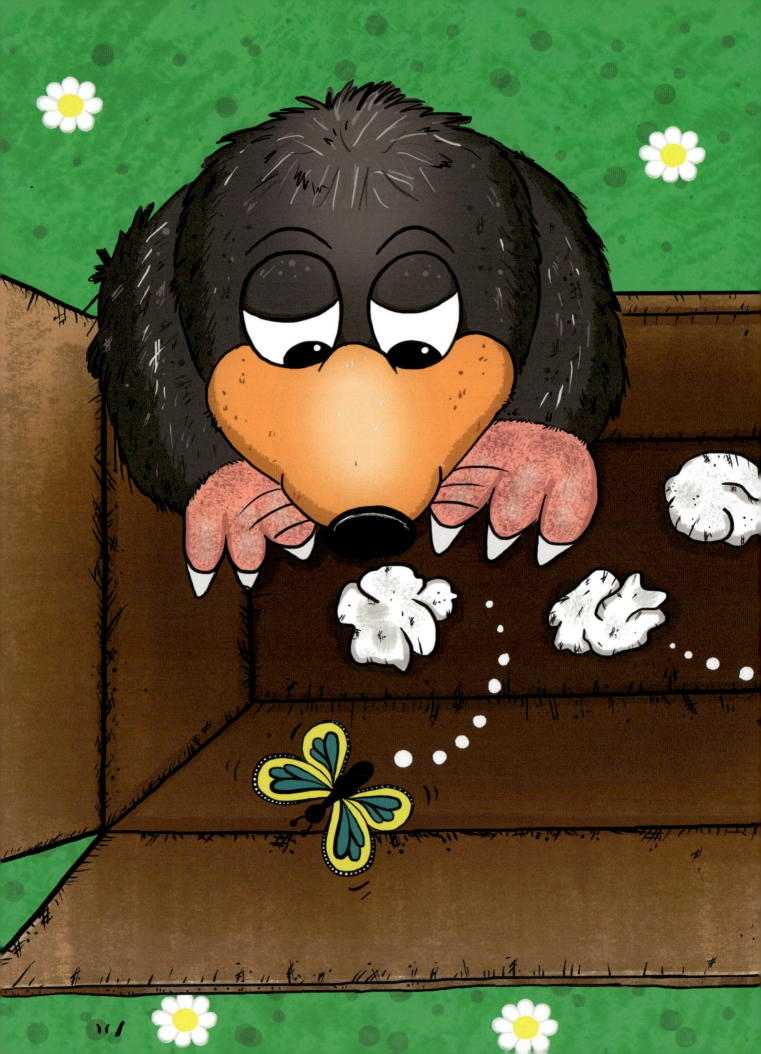

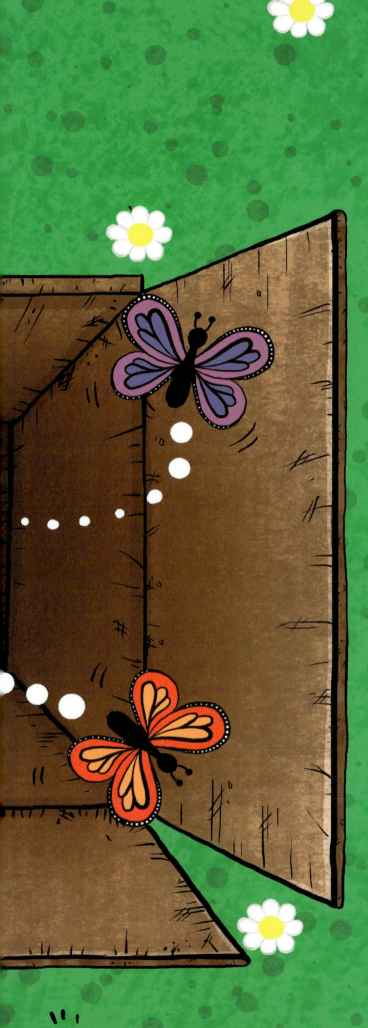
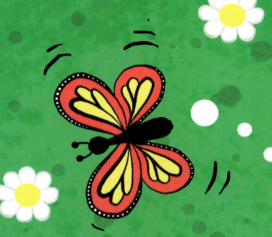

He asked his good friend Oscar the Owl, if he could look in the box at the butterflies, and found most of them had flown away.

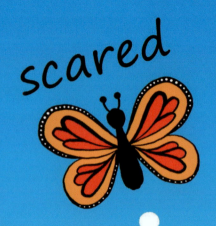 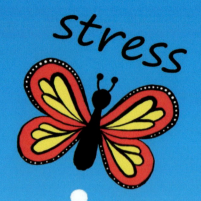

"Why was I worrying about that, when it didn't even happen?"

worry

upset

nervous

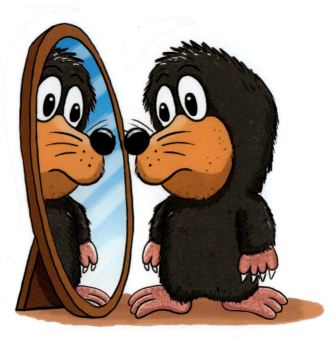

# 1. Identify

What makes you worry? Worrying makes me sad. Worrying makes me feel alone.

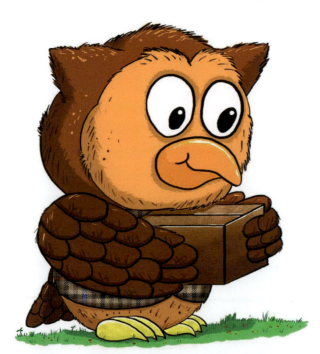

# 2. Support

Talk to someone who you trust. Share your worries with a good friend or a grown up.

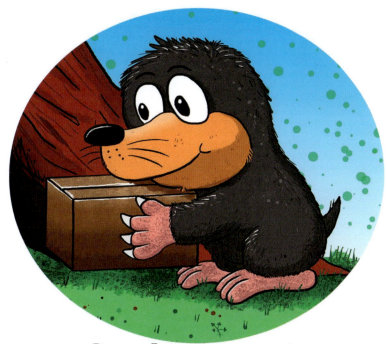

# 3. Accept

I don't like feeling like this. I want someone to help me. I want my worries to go away.

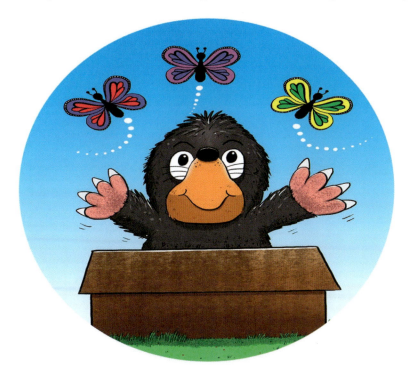

# 4. Let Go!

Write your worries down. Let someone else take care of your worries. Do something that makes you happy.

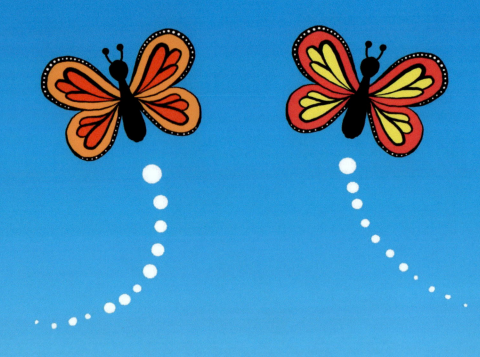

Text copyright  Lyndsey Griffin-Cowap 2019

Illustration copyright  Mark Lloyd 2019

ISBN 9781071089569

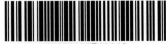
46989160R00019

Printed in Poland
by Amazon Fulfillment
Poland Sp. z o.o., Wrocław